W9-DAJ-533

WITHDRAWN
from N. F. Bourke Memorial Library
Cayuga County Community College

NORMAN F. BOURKE
MEMORIAL LIBRARY
CAYUGA COMMUNITY
COLLEGE
AUBURN, NEW YORK

STEROIDS

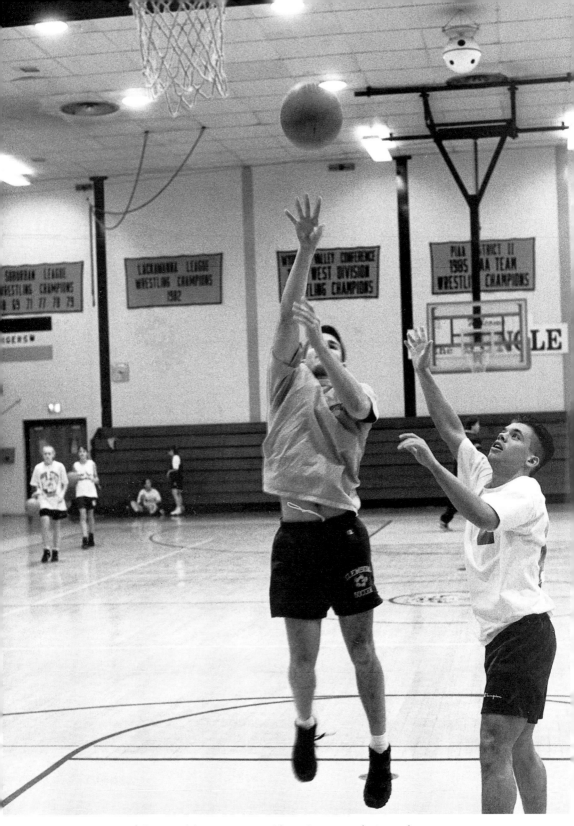

Some athletes use steroids to improve their performance.

THE DRUG ABUSE PREVENTION LIBRARY

STEROIDS

Lawrence Clayton, Ph.D.

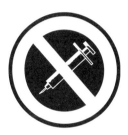

THE ROSEN PUBLISHING GROUP, INC.

NEW YORK

The people pictured in this book are only models. They in no way practice or endorse the activities illustrated. Captions serve only to explain the subjects of photographs and do not in any way imply a connection between the real-life models and the staged situations.

To
Larry, my son,
a great drug-free athlete

Published in 1996, 1999 by The Rosen Publishing Group, Inc., 29 East 21st Street, New York, NY 10010

Copyright © 1996, 1999 by The Rosen Publishing Group, Inc.

All rights reserved. No part of this book may be reproduced in any form without permission in writing from the publisher, except by a reviewer.

Revised Edition

Library of Congress Cataloging-in-Publication Data

Clayton, L. (Lawrence)
    Steroids / Lawrence Clayton. — 1st ed.
        p. cm. — (The Drug abuse prevention library)
    Includes bibliographical references (p.) and index.
    ISBN 0-8239-2888-8
    1. Doping in sports—Juvenile literature.
    2. Anabolic steroids—Health aspects—Juvenile literature. I. Title. II. Series.
    RC1230.C538 1999
    613.8—dc20   95-1464
                                                       CIP
                                                       AC

Manufactured in the United States of America

Contents

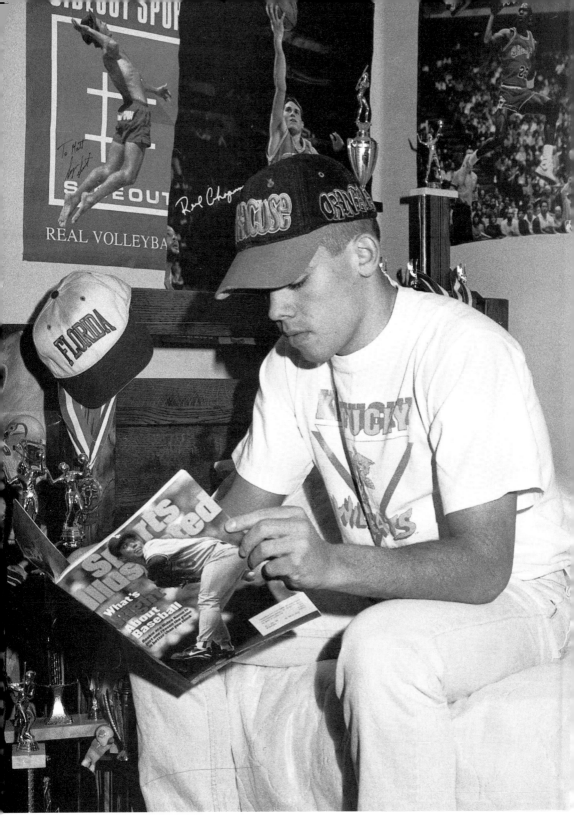

Sports are very important to many people.

CHAPTER 1

The Value of Sports

What do sports mean to you? Evenings spent glued to the television for the World Series? Weeks spent building up to the NBA final? A month spent watching the World Cup? Or you may participate in sports.

Sports play an important part in the social life of many teens. Some wear their favorite baseball player's jersey. Some kids constantly read the sports section of the newspaper. Others plaster their walls with posters, pictures, and photos of their favorite teams or players.

If you are more than an armchair fan, you may try to see your favorite team, or your local team, as often as possible. You may join friends to watch your favorite teams on television or tune in to hear sports commentary on the radio. You may

8 even help coach a team.

Today young people participate in more sports—baseball, basketball, football, hockey, martial arts, soccer, softball, track and field—than ever before. They start younger too. The average age for beginners is just over five.

Sports mean different things to different people, and different sports appeal to different kinds of people. If you are an athlete, you may be part of a team or involved in an individual sport. In either case, sports offer you the opportunity to learn the importance of loyalty, sportsmanship, and teamwork.

Sports and Loyalty

Even in sports in which you perform as an individual, such as track and field or tennis, you are usually part of a team. As part of a team you develop a sense of loyalty to things that are larger than you. It is not just a team; it is *your* team. You talk about "we" instead of "I," and you come to care about the success of the group, not just your own wins and losses.

Sports and Teamwork

Loyalty and teamwork go hand in hand. The teamwork that you learn on the field is the teamwork that you will need all through life. Teamwork means that although everyone is recognized as an individual, the success of the group is the ultimate goal.

Teamwork builds cars, bridges, televisions, computers, and schools. Learning to work together with others toward a common goal is essential, and sports helps.

Sports and Fair Play

Sports also teach about fair play. When you were little, you didn't understand the idea of fair play. You wanted what you wanted when you wanted it and didn't care about fairness. Fair play is getting what you deserve when you deserve it.

Fair play means not cheating. Fair play means whoever is the faster, sharper, more disciplined player is the winner. You know how you feel if people are given a reward for something because of whom they know, not their ability. Similarly, you learn that it is cheating if you are rewarded for something that somebody else should have won.

Sports and Sportsmanship

You play and you win. You play and you

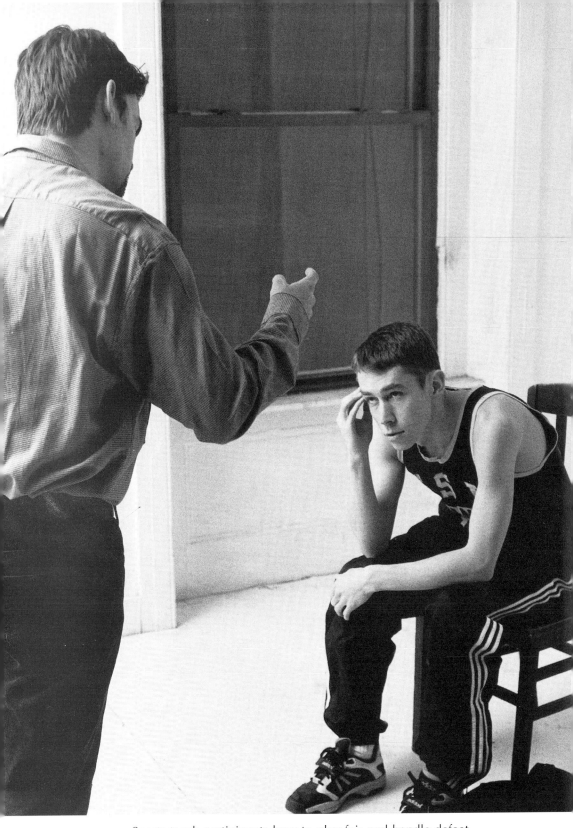

Sports teach participants how to play fair and handle defeat.

lose. But you keep playing. Sportsmanship is about being a good loser and an
honorable winner. Good sportsmanship is
about shaking hands with your opponent
after a game.

When you lose the game you don't
lose your temper. You learn to take a
knockdown and to get up without retali-
ating. You may have lost this time, but
you learn from your mistakes and use
that to your advantage next time.

The lessons you learn about sportsmanship will carry you through the rest
of your life. You will not always get the
things that you hope for. Life is full of
disappointments. But when you don't get
that job, or that apartment, or that date,
good sportsmanship will help.

Sports and the Family

In many families parents encourage their
kids to play sports. They are happy to
see you do well, but if you don't win,
they support you. Your parents have
probably already learned about sportsmanship, and they know that playing the
game is more important than who wins
or loses.

However, some parents are less con-
cerned with sportsmanship. They want

12 | their kids to win, win, win. They are the proudest parents if their teens perform well. But they are cold and distant or angry if their teenager drops the ball, misses the play, or strikes out. For their children, the pressure to succeed at all costs—so that they don't disappoint their parents—is very strong. The pressure can cause them to turn to drugs to enhance their performance.

Sports and Drugs

Sports are such an important part of young people's lives that it is not surprising that some athletes try using drugs to become better athletes. They may believe that drug use is a shortcut to fame, glory, and success.

One category of drugs that are abused by athletes are steroids. They can make an athlete run faster or be stronger in the short term. But an athlete who uses them cheats himself or herself, and breaks the rules of fair competition. In the long term, such an athlete may also end up in the hospital, a juvenile detention center, or even an early grave.

CHAPTER 2

A Short History of Steroid Abuse

*I*n July 1988, a subcommittee of the Judiciary Committee of the U.S. House of Representatives held a hearing on crime. This body hears only issues of the most serious national importance. But there they were, our Representatives and experts from around the country—sports doctors, coaches, athletes, and representatives of the National Football League (NFL), the International Olympic Committee (IOC), the American Medical Association (AMA), the National Collegiate Athletic Association (NCAA), and many more—discussing steroid abuse.

The NFL representative read a statement that said in part, "Anabolic steroids are well worth congressional concern. It

14 | has become clear that they pose numerous and serious medical risks."

Dr. William Howard, chief physician at the Sports Medicine Clinic of Union Memorial Hospital, said that as many as 50 percent of professional athletes were taking steroids to enhance their performance.

Some were even taking steroids that were intended only for race horses. Several were taking twice the amount that would be medically safe for a horse. They were making themselves sick, and some had died.

The Strange Beginnings

How did this happen? How did steroid abuse reach such unhealthy levels?

It started in a most peculiar way. In 1771, John Hunter transplanted the testes of a rooster into a hen. The result was that the hen became more "rooster-like" in appearance and behavior.

The next experiment was more than 100 years later, in 1889, when Dr. Charles E. Brown-Sequard injected himself with testicular extract. He reported feeling stronger and smarter and having improved digestion.

In 1935, scientists discovered that

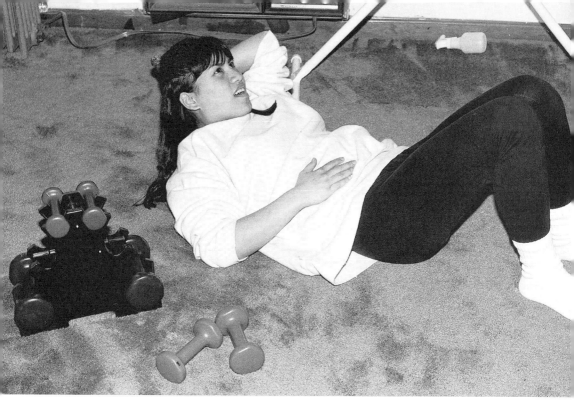

Athletes may try steroids when they feel that physical training isn't enough.

testosterone was the chemical that caused males to be male. From then on, people were interested in finding out just how strong testosterone could make a person.

The idea that drugs could enhance performance was not new. Athletes had been using amphetamines (speed) and other drugs for this purpose for many years, and there had been many casualties.

A Dutch cyclist died in 1986 after being doped with cocaine and heroin by his coach. This caused several sporting organizations to require athletes to be examined for drugs by doctors.

15

16 | *Athletes Join the Parade*

Weight lifters from the former Soviet Union began using steroids in 1950. Because of this, they dominated all weight-lifting competition for many years. In 1954, the United States Olympic team's physician, Dr. John B. Ziegler, gave steroids to his team, hoping to help them compete with the Soviets.

By 1957, drug use was so widespread that the American Medical Association (AMA) established a group now called the Committee on the Medical Aspects of Sports in a vain attempt to control athletes' drug abuse. Other countries followed suit.

Despite this, a Danish cyclist died at the 1960 Olympic Games from use of amphetamines. In 1967, a French and an English cyclist died from drug abuse. This caused the IOC to begin testing athletes for drugs. In one year, eight cyclists in Winnipeg, two cyclists in Rome, and 17 percent of the Italian soccer team tested positive for drugs.

When drug testing was announced at the world championships in 1970, one athlete dropped out immediately and three others tested positive. At the World Weight-Lifting Championships that year, nine weight lifters were tested; eight showed evidence of drug use.

Olympic Drug Tests

In 1972, the IOC began full-scale drug testing. As a result, four athletes lost medals they had won, and seven others were banned from the Games forever.

Anabolic steroids were officially banned by the IOC in 1975. Even so, the next year two male weight lifters and one female discus thrower were disqualified. Eight others were banned that summer in Montreal. In 1983, the IOC added caffeine and testosterone to the list of banned substances, and the U.S. Food and Drug Administration banned the production of Dianabol (a steroid). Diuretics (drugs to increase the output of urine) and certain forms of corticosteroids were added to the list of banned chemicals in 1985.

Brian Bosworth, All-American defensive back of the University of Oklahoma, was banned from postseason play for steroid abuse by the NCAA in 1986. The next year, the NFL checked for steroids and gave a thirty-day suspension to anyone who tested positive.

In May 1987, the U.S. Department of Justice filed 100-count indictments

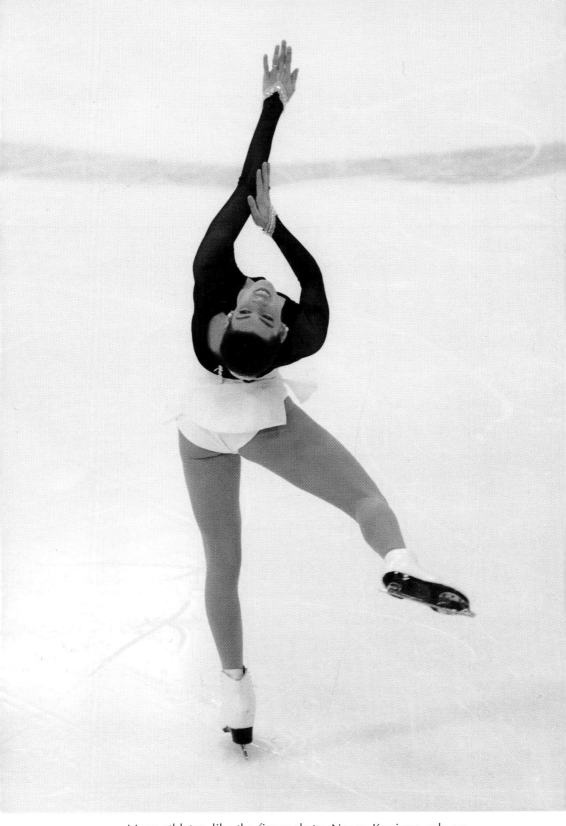

Many athletes, like the figure skater Nancy Kerrigan, rely on their natural strength and talent and stay drug-free.

against thirty-four persons for sale and distribution of anabolic steroids. In the same year, the IOC discovered that some athletes were still using steroids during the off-season, so they began "out-of-competition" drug testing.

At the 1988 Summer Olympics, the world's fastest runner, Canadian Ben Johnson, won a gold medal but was stripped of it and ousted from the Games after he tested positive for steroids.

Steroid Epidemic

By that time, it was clear that a new drug epidemic had struck. It was also clear that it was fueled by anabolic steroids.

That is how the U.S. House of Representatives got involved. At the end of the hearing, steroids were placed under the same restrictions as heroin and cocaine.

Despite this, in 1989 the National Institute on Drug Abuse (NIDA) reported that adolescent steroid use had risen to 4.7 percent of males and 1.3 percent of females. A year later, the U.S. Inspector General reported that adolescent abuse of steroids continued to climb to 11 percent of males and 3 percent of females. That is about 500,000 teenagers. The NCAA

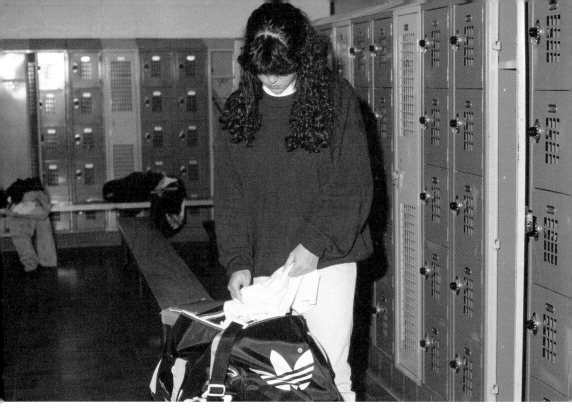

Steroid abuse occurs among both male and female athletes.

joined the IOC in performing intensive drug testing of its athletes.

The Anabolic Steroids Control Act of 1990 set severe penalties for both sale and possession of steroids. The fine for sale was set at $250,000 for the first offense and $500,000 for the second offense. Simple possession can carry a $1,000 fine.

Today, the NIDA estimates that more than 1 million adolescents are steroid users. They support a $100 million trade in black market steroids.

CHAPTER 3

Types of Steroids

*T*he human body contains some 600 different steroids, but there are only three main types. This chapter discusses the medical use and the abuse potential of each type of steroid.

Corticosteroids
Corticosteroids are medically used to control inflammation and pain. They have little potential for abuse.

Estrogenic Steroids
These steroids are made from the female sex hormone estrogen and are used for birth control and as estrogen replacement after the ovaries have been removed or

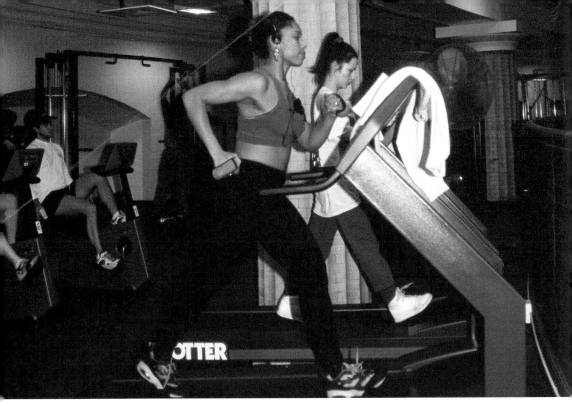

Anabolic steroids, which build muscle tone, have a high potential for abuse.

ceased functioning. They have no potential for abuse.

Anabolic Steroids

Anabolic steroids are made from the male sex hormone (testosterone) and are used medically, *in limited dosages*, for patients with diseases such as cancer or AIDS. They increase muscle and tendon strength for patients who cannot recover naturally. They have an extremely high potential for abuse.

People use anabolic steroids to build muscle and enhance their performance. It might take a teenage boy a year of intensive weight lifting to add thirty pounds of muscle to his body. Anabolic steroids, taken in huge amounts, can do it in twelve weeks. Of course, the side effects can be deadly.

The chart below gives the generic and brand names of some of the most common anabolic steroids and how each is administered.

Common Anabolic Steroids

Generic Name	Brand Name	Administration
Calusterone	Methosarb	Oral
Danazol	Danocrine, Danol, Cyclomen, Danatrol, Danobrin, Ladogar, Winobanin	Oral
Dromostandolone	Masteril, Masterone, (Drostanolone) Metormon	Injectable
Proplonate	Permastril, Drolban	Oral
Ethylestrenol	Maxibolin, Orabolin, Otgabolin	
Fluoxymesterone	Android-F, Halotestin, Oralsterone, Oratestin, Ora-Testryl, Ultandren	Oral
Formebolone	Esiclene, Hubernol	Injectable
Furazabol	Miotolone	Oral and Injectable
Mebolazine	Roxilon	Oral
Mesterolone	Mestoranum, Proviron	Oral
Methandriol	Sinsex, Stenediol, Troformone	Oral

24	Generic Name	Brand Name	Administration
	Methandrostenolone (Methandienone)	Andoredan, Danabol, Dianabol, Encephan, Lanabolin, Metabolina, Metaboline, Metanabol, Metastenol, Nerobol, Perbolin	Oral and Injectable
	Methenolone	Primobolan, Primobolan Despot, Primobolan S, Primonbol	Oral and Injectable
	Methyltestosterone	Androyd, Glosso-Sterandryl, Mesteron, Metandren, Neo-Hombreol, Neohombreol-M, Methyltestosterone Orchisterone, Oreton, Methyl, Primotest, Testin, Testomet, Testovis, Testred, Virilon, Virormone-Oral	Oral
	Mibolerone	Nilevar	Oral
	Nandrolone	Anobolin LA-100, Androlone Hybolin Deconoate, Kabolin, Nandrolin, Neo-Durabolic	Injectable
	Oxabolone	Steranabol Despot, Steranabol Ritardo	Injectable
	Oxandrolone	Anavar, Antitriol, Lonavar	Oral
	Oxymesterone	Anamidol, Balinmax, Oranabol, Oranabol-10	Oral
	Oxymetholone	Anapolon-50, Androl 50, Adroyd,	Oral

Generic Name	Brand Name	Administration	*25*
	Anadroyd, Anasterone, Anasteronal Nastenon, Oxitosona-50, Pardroyd, Plenastril, Synasteron, Zenalosyn		
Quinbolone	Anabolicum Vister	Oral	
Stanozolol	Wnstrol, Anasyth, Stromba, Strombajeck, Winstrol	Oral	
Testosterone	Androil, Anadronate, BayTestone, Depo-Testosterone, Jectatest-LA, Malogen LA, Sustanon, Restandol, Testate, Testone LA, Testostroval	Oral and Injectable	
Trenbolone	Parabolan, Finajet, Finaplix	Injectable	

These drugs are available only by prescription. Some, such as Dianabol, are used only for animals and are not available even by prescription.

Drug dealers do a huge black market business selling anabolic steroids. In the early 1990s the U.S. Food and Drug Administration estimated that $600,000 worth of all illegal steroid sales take place through private fitness centers and

26 | gymnasiums every year. That's about 79 percent of all the steroids sold in the United States.

CHAPTER 4

Steroids Can Damage Your Body

*W*hen anabolic steroids are used by doctors, they help heal and increase strength. But when they are abused they are dangerous. Like most drugs, they have side effects. Because anabolic steroids are made primarily from the male hormone testosterone, the side effects are different for boys and girls.

While steroids may help a runner win a race, in the long term they will cause him or her great losses. When a person stops taking steroids, the strength that the steroids gave that person fades away. The dangerous side effects are usually permanent. Steroid abuse can irreversibly damage your body.

Side Effects That Can Strike Boys

Steroid abuse makes males look more like females. It causes unusual breast development, and shrinking and drying up of the testicles.

Other side effects are swelling of the prostate gland to the point of needing to be catheterized (process in which a hollow tube is used to drain fluids) to urinate, and impotence. Severe penis pain can occur too.

Side Effects That Can Strike Girls

Steroid abuse makes females look more like males. It causes girls to grow facial and body hair and develop male-pattern baldness. Steroid abuse also deepens the voice, causes menstrual problems, and can result in clitoral enlargement.

In pregnant women, use of steroids can result in devastating birth defects that have lifelong effects on the child.

Side Effects That Can Strike Anyone

Everyone's body is unique, and each responds to drugs in its own way. Following are several possible side effects of steroid abuse. Although you will not develop every one of these problems if you choose to abuse steroids, you will experience many of the side effects.

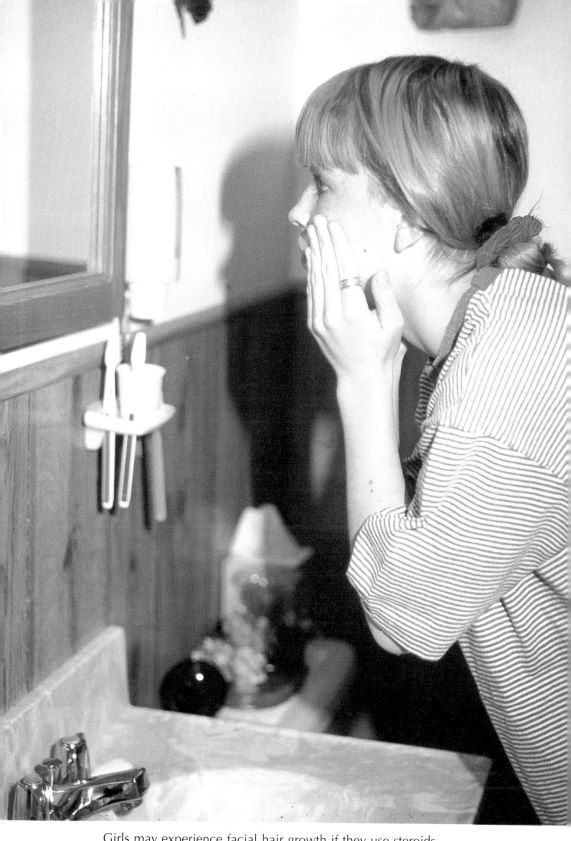

Girls may experience facial hair growth if they use steroids.

30 | ## *Skin Problems*

Steroid abuse wreaks havoc with the skin, the body's largest organ. It causes:

Extremely oily skin. People who use steroids often look as if they've been working at an auto lubrication station, because their clothes get so oily. Any dirt in the air sticks to them, and by the end of the day ring-around-the-collar is very evident.

Hives. Many people have an allergic reaction to steroids that causes hives, a horribly itchy rash. Some people also get purple spots on the head, neck, and body.

Severe acne. Teenagers are subject to acne, but steroid abusers get a very severe kind that is deep below the surface of the skin. It often becomes inflamed and erupts into huge pus- and blood-filled pimples that take a long time to heal. When they do heal, they frequently leave permanent scars on a person's face, neck, chest, and back.

Coronary Artery Problems

Steroids cause changes in the body that set the abuser up for coronary artery problems. A blood analysis often looks as if it came from someone very old. It shows high levels of everything bad—high blood pressure, high cholesterol, high levels of sugar and fat cells. Steroids also weaken the heart, which leads to such problems as heart attack, stroke, and premature senility. Most steroid abusers die long before they should.

Petra Kind Schneider is a swimmer from the former East Germany. She is famous for her performance in the 400-meter individual medley. Schneider now suffers from heart and liver problems because of past steroid abuse. She says steroids were administered to her as "little blue pills" when she was fourteen.

Liver and Kidney Problems

Steroids are particularly hard on the liver, making it unable to clear the blood of poisons. This causes jaundice, a yellowing of the eyes and skin. It also frequently causes liver tumors.

Steroids attack the kidneys, causing them to malfunction and eventually fail. As the kidneys grow weaker, they are unable to do their job of eliminating excess water from the body. This water retention gives steroid abusers a bloated look and causes their legs and feet to swell.

Muscle and Bone Problems

The liver, kidney, and heart problems caused by steroids eventually cause the muscles to cramp painfully. Muscle and tendon injuries become frequent. Bones begin to ache in various parts of the body.

A problem that is especially damaging to teenagers is premature maturation; that is, the body becomes mature before it should. A twelve-year-old may develop large muscles and a beard and start going bald. Growth plates in his bones close forever so that he can never grow taller. By the time he's fourteen, all the other boys are bigger and stronger. By the time he's sixteen, he is too small to compete at all.

Internal Problems

Steroids mess up the internal organ systems. Abusers often feel nauseated and sometimes vomit blood. They have diarrhea, chills, tongue pain, and permanent bad breath.

They may experience fainting, dizziness, and fatigue. Steroids can also cause blood poisoning, gallstones, and cancer.

Other Complications

Steroid abuse can cause epileptic-like seizures (uncontrolled, involuntary con-

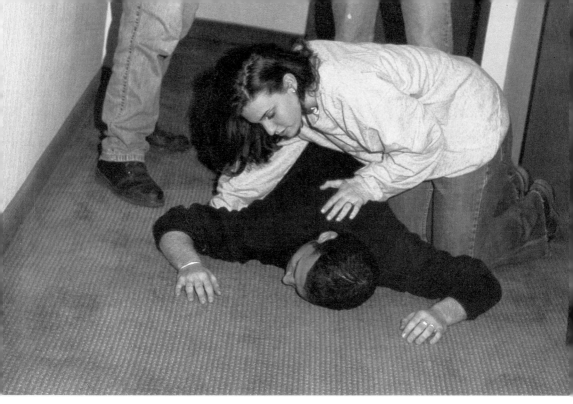

Steroid abusers may suffer from seizures.

vulsions), which sometimes result in death. Most abusers suffer insomnia (inability to sleep) and severe headaches.

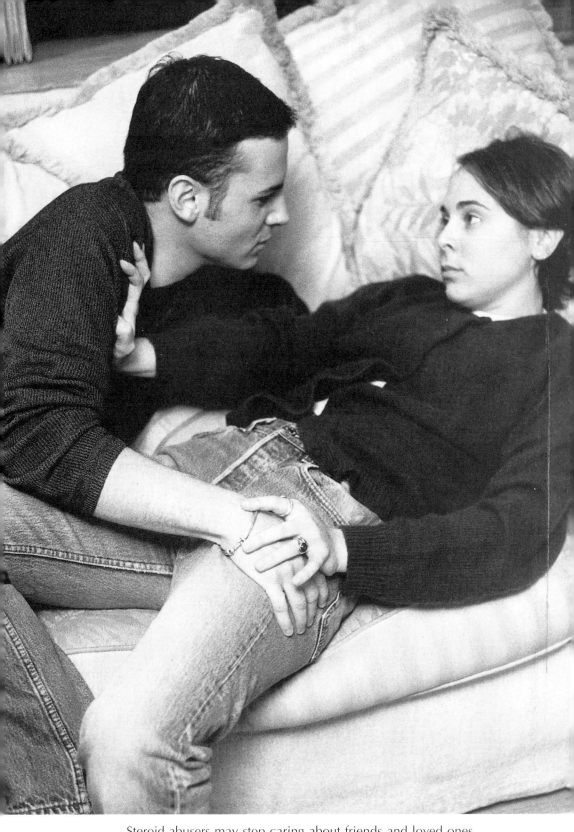

Steroid abusers may stop caring about friends and loved ones.

CHAPTER 5

Steroids Can Change Your Personality

Steroids change your personality in very specific ways, all of them undesirable. Some are so dangerous that they could cost you your life or cause you to take someone else's.

Steroids can make you self-centered, egotistical, and inconsiderate. They can make you angry, aggressive, and violent— perhaps homicidal. They make some people depressed and even suicidal.

Steroids Can Make You Self-Centered

Steroids mess up your mind. Users become "stuck on themselves." Little by little, family, friends, teammates—even girlfriends or boyfriends—mean less and less to them. Eventually they can reach the point where only their own desires

36 are important. Other people become just things to use to make the abuser happy.

Brick

Brick was called Brick because he was so much bigger and stronger than everyone else. In his junior year, Brick was quarterback for the school team and the most popular guy with all the girls. He was good-looking, strong, and friendly, and he always had a good word to say. He also had a supportive ear to lend to his teammates. His friend Henry also played football, but he wasn't as serious about it.

In the summer before senior year, Brick decided that he wanted to make the state football team. Henry decided to try too, and he began to take it more seriously. They trained together every day. Although they were friends and both were good, Henry seemed to be doing better. Brick began to worry that Henry would get chosen but he wouldn't. Brick started taking steroids to improve his chances.

At first, it seemed to work. Brick put on weight and was faster and stronger than ever. His coach was impressed with his performance and so were his teammates. But that wasn't enough for Brick. He still wanted to make the state team. That was his dream, and nothing was going to stop him from fulfilling it.

One week before the trials, Brick and

Henry were still training together. Brick was much stronger, but he was still threatened by Henry's natural ability. Brick and Henry planned to run along the river together the next morning.

That night Brick sneaked out of his house and went down to the river. He dug a hole along the running path and covered it with branches and leaves, then went home to sleep. When he was out running with Henry the next morning, he made sure that Henry ran on the side where the hole was. Unsuspecting, Henry stepped into the hole and severely twisted his ankle. He was unable to play football for several weeks, and he wasn't able to try out for the state team.

Brick went to the state tryouts. He did not know that the tryouts included a drug test. Brick failed the test. He returned home to face his family, coach, teammates, and friends.

Brick was thrown off his school team. Instead of finding success through taking steroids, as he had hoped, he lost all chance of reaching his dream.

Steroid abuse seriously damages your ability to care about others. Many steroid abusers report feeling very alone. They become self-centered and insensitive.

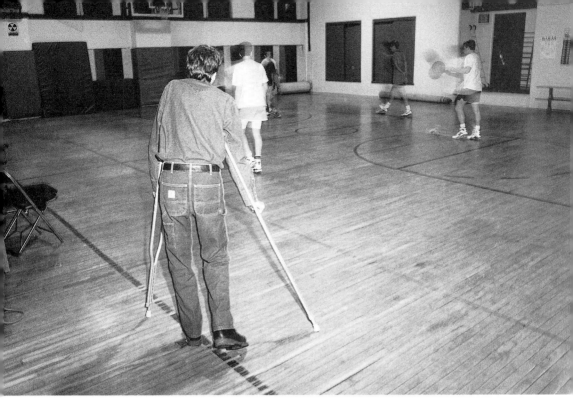
As well as causing physical problems, steroids can make athletes angry and violent.

Steroids Can Make You Angry

Another way steroids mess with your mind is that they cause you to be unreasonably angry—sometimes at those you most love, sometimes at total strangers. For some, the consequences are serious, even life-threatening.

Rita

Rita was the best 800-meter runner that her school had seen in years. But that was not enough for Rita. She wanted to be more than just the school record holder. She wanted to take her running career as far as it could go.

Rita was also a member of a local running team. At one of her club meetings she noticed a woman talking and laughing with the club president. The woman watched Rita run and could see that she had talent. At the end of the meeting the woman approached Rita and told her how talented she was. Rita was very flattered. The woman also told Rita that she could be even more successful.

"How?" asked Rita. "I train as hard as I can."

"Try these," the woman said, and handed her a packet. "They're steroids. But that's just between you and me, okay?" And the woman left.

Rita carried the pills around for a week. She'd heard that steroids were bad for you, but her desire to improve her performance made her want to try them. She took the steroids. She kept to her usual training schedule, and she noticed a rapid improvement in her speed and strength. Everyone was impressed by Rita's increasing ability. But she found that she was also more irritable.

One day in June, Rita was playing volleyball with her friends at the beach when a fight broke out.

"Martha, what are you doing?" yelled Rita, snatching the ball out of Martha's hands. "It's not your serve."

"It is. Give me the ball!" Martha yelled

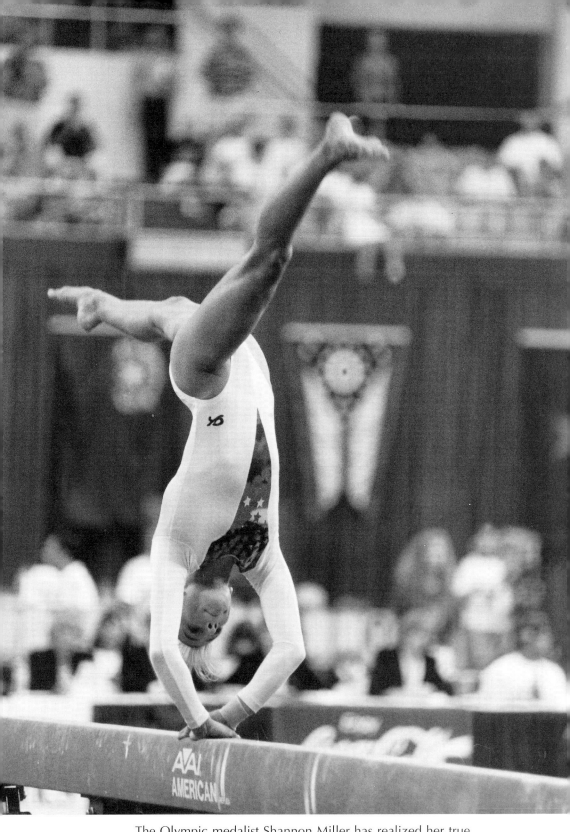

The Olympic medalist Shannon Miller has realized her true
potential without help from drugs.

back. The disagreement escalated, with **41** *Martha and Rita shouting back and forth at each other. Suddenly Rita, in a rage, took off over the dunes to the parking lot. She got into her car and drove wildly through the lot, sideswiping parked cars as she did. She caused thousands of dollars' worth of damage. Then she drove away. Later, she couldn't believe what she had done.*

Anger is a common side effect of steroid abuse. It cost Rita her friends and thousands of dollars. Instead of reacting as she usually would have, Rita realized, chemicals in her body were deciding her reactions for her.

Steroids Make You Violent

People who abuse steroids can become violent in a flash. This makes them unpredictable and untrustworthy. Having steroid abusers as friends can be dangerous and perhaps deadly.

Sherry

Sherry had never felt like part of the crowd. She felt alone, left out. She wanted desperately to be popular.

She would have liked to play sports, but she thought she was too short and small to be

*any good. "I'll never be good at anything,"
she told herself.*

*Then one day Shannon Miller, the
Olympic medalist, spoke to the student body
during assembly.*

*Right away Sherry liked her. Shannon
was short, just like her. When she talked
about her life, she said that she had always
felt left out but that gymnastics had changed
all that. Now Sherry knew exactly what she
would do. Gymnastics could change her life
the way it had changed Shannon's.*

*That very day, Sherry enrolled in a gym-
nastics class. She found she was too weak to
do well, especially in her ankles. Then a
"friend" from class introduced her to steroids.
She started getting stronger. But her temper
became more violent.*

*A year later, Sherry was a much stronger
gymnast. There was even talk of putting her
on the team. Sherry was delighted. "You need
more work on the balance beam, Sherry,"
said Cindy, another gymnast. "You'll never
make the team like that."*

*Sherry's face turned red and she
shouted, "I'm better than you!"*

"I was only trying to help," said Cindy.

*Sherry began screaming and cursing. "You
jerk, who appointed you God?" Then Sherry
hit her in the face. Not once, but over and*

over. She was like a wild person. It took the **43**
*coach and several other athletes to subdue
her. Cindy had to be hospitalized.*

*Sherry was suspended from school. Three
days later, when she showed up for practice
the coach said, "Sherry, we don't need you
here. Go get some help."*

"Roid rage" has been known to cause some steroid abusers to commit murder. The girl Sherry attacked was lucky to be alive. And Sherry was lucky that she didn't go to jail.

Steroids Can Make You Depressed

Abuse of steroids is so hard on the body that the abuser eventually has to stop using them or die. But those who do stop often become seriously depressed. Mental health professionals call this kind of depression steroid-induced anhedonia. It means a period of time when everything loses its meaning and joy: sports, friends, family, being big and strong, even life itself. It could also be called steroid withdrawal. By whatever name, it is horrible to experience.

Randy

*Randy had secretly been taking steroids for
two years to improve his ability as a sprinter.*

44 | *He was fast and strong, but he was experiencing side effects from the steroids. He had acne, and his bones often ached. Randy was also throwing up blood.*

He was terrified and did not know what to do. His first reaction was to tell his mother, but he did not want to scare her, so he went to the school nurse and told her everything. She was not judgmental about his drug taking, but she did tell him that he would have to stop taking steroids immediately.

The nurse had seen cases like Randy's before. She advised him that he would probably have some withdrawal symptoms, and that he should tell his parents so that they could help him. Armed with a book about steroids, and some help-line phone numbers, Randy returned home.

He told his mother about his two-year abuse of steroids. Naturally she was very upset, but she contacted the school nurse herself and read the book that Randy had brought home. When she found Randy sitting on the end of his bed every morning too depressed even to get dressed and go to school, she was able to help and support him. She took him to a therapist who was familiar with the effects of steroids and equipped to deal with Randy's withdrawal symptoms.

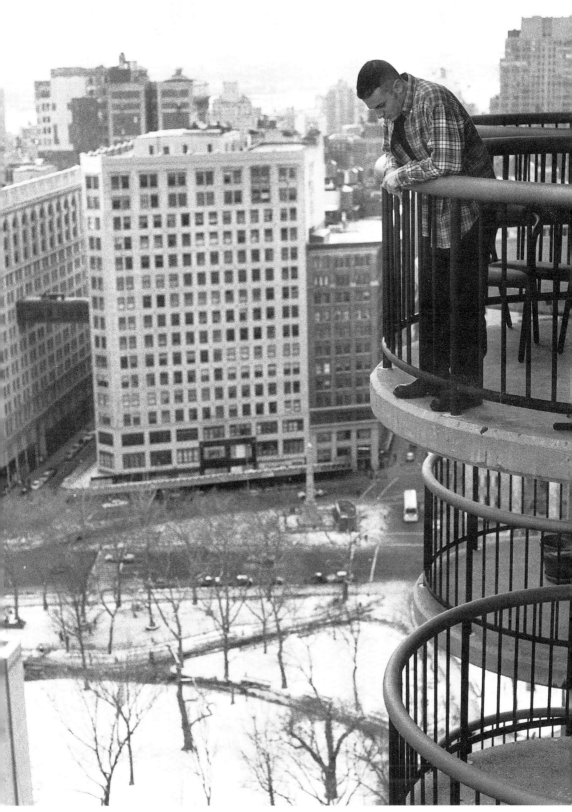

Depression caused by steroid withdrawal can lead some
former users to commit suicide.

46 Randy suffered deep depression for many months, but he gradually stopped vomiting blood. With the help and support of his mother, the school nurse, and drug-abuse support groups, he was able to return to being a healthy teenager.

When steroid abusers decide to quit taking drugs, it helps if they seek medical assistance. A school nurse or even a school counselor can give teens advice and support. When a person stops taking a drug and goes through withdrawal, he or she needs all the support and information available.

Steroids Can Make You Suicidal

Some steroid abusers don't get over their use. The depression is so severe that they just can't cope, and they end up taking their own lives.

Vernice

Vernice was on the basketball team. She was a real team player, and she played well. Her school team, Central High, were finalists in the state championships every year. They were setting new standards for women's basketball and were proud of their achievements. Vernice knew she was not the only girl on the team who was taking steroids, but nobody ever discussed it. Steroids were not allowed and were kept a secret. Vernice did not tell her parents that she used steroids.

One day, Vernice vomited blood. She felt pain in her belly. She went to the school nurse and took some tests. She learned that she had liver damage. The nurse told her that it was not too severe, and that if she stopped taking the drugs now it would not get any worse. Vernice was relieved.

The nurse also recommended that Vernice become part of a drug rehabilitation program to get over the steroids. Vernice worried when she heard that. She did not want to tell her parents, especially her father, who was so proud of her achievements. She decided to try quitting steroids on her own. This was a brave choice, but it was difficult.

Although the nurse had given Vernice material to read about steroids and steroid withdrawal, she was not prepared for the effects she experienced.

Soon after she quit taking the steroids she began feeling depressed as a result of withdrawal. At the same time her performance on the court began to deteriorate noticeably.

When her coach came to her and asked if she was having problems or was not feeling well, she said no. She was afraid to admit to the coach that she had been taking steroids, because she knew he would not approve and could remove her from the team.

Vernice's coach thought that she might be experiencing personal problems. He wanted to empathize, but it was nearing the end of the season. He could not afford to have a weak player on the team. Vernice was dropped from the basketball team just one month before the state championships.

Vernice was devastated. She had already been feeling depressed. Now she felt hopeless, alone, and miserable. For days she did not talk to anyone. Her family was worried. They had never seen her like this before.

Vernice went out for a bike ride one afternoon to try to feel better. She rode several miles to where the town gave way to the country. It was a beautiful day. When she reached the river, she came to a sudden stop in the middle of the bridge. Vernice got off her bike and leaned it against the railing of the bridge. She looked at the river for a long time, then climbed up onto the railing.

She felt so depressed and helpless that she considered throwing herself into the water below. Fortunately, a woman driving by noticed her and called for help. Someone arrived in time to talk Vernice down and save her life. After that, Vernice told her parents what had happened. They helped her find

help to get her through her depression. They
surprised Vernice: they were very supportive.

A year later, Vernice was feeling much better. She had gotten back on the basketball team. She was still a team player—and she went with her team to the state championships.

Vernice was fortunate and found help. Eventually she began to feel like herself again.

Even though the worst of the depression associated with withdrawal is usually over in three to six months, steroid-induced anhedonia can last as long as five years.

CHAPTER 6

People Who Can Help

*I*f you are young and involved in sports, you may have been offered or may even be taking steroids. But steroids are dangerous. They give you a short-term boost in body strength and power, but in the long term they will cause your body harm.

If you or someone you know wants to quit, it is important to seek medical supervision. You have been chemically altering your body. Now it has to go through further changes. Following are some places where you can get help.

School Nurse

School nurses are trained to look out for drug abuse. They understand the reasons

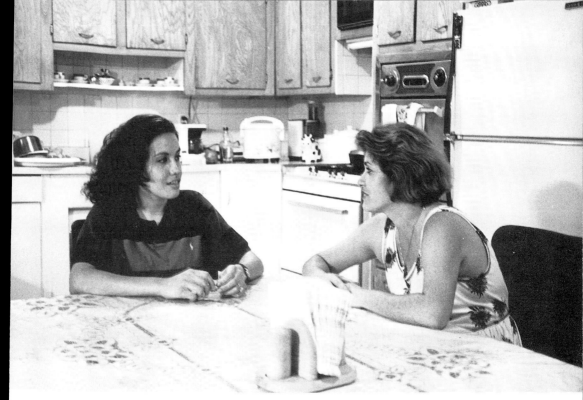

Give your parents a chance to help you kick a steroid habit.

why you chose to take steroids, and they can help you to quit. Nurses will not be shocked by what they see or hear. No matter how ashamed you are of yourself, they will have seen worse.

The nurse's office is a good place to start in your attempt to quit using steroids. He or she can provide you with plenty of information to take home to your parents. A nurse can also connect you with the places you will need to go for further help.

Parents

Most parents care deeply about their

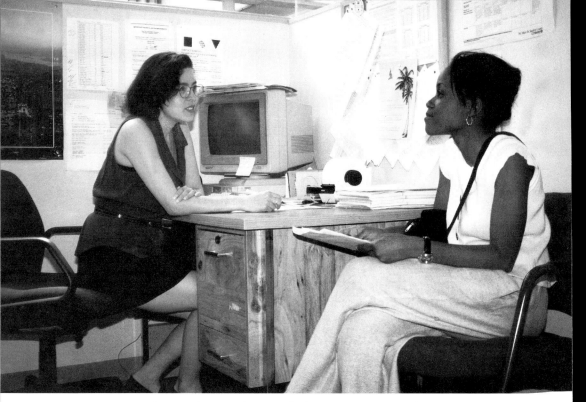

Professional counselors can help users overcome their addiction.

Certified Alcohol and Drug Counselor (CADC)

CADCs are the professionals in the drug and alcohol field. They spend much of their lives helping people who are addicted. They can help you in more ways than almost anyone else.

CADCs are trained to counsel persons who are addicted. They can help you talk to your parents about the problem. They can also help you decide what steps to take to overcome your addiction.

If you are going into withdrawal, they will recognize the symptoms and get you the help you need. Because they have treated many other young people who are addicted, they can tell you what to expect as you take the steps to stop using steroids.

To find a CADC, look in the Yellow Pages under Alcoholism or Drug Counselors. You will find the letters CADC after the counselors' names.

Your Doctor

Another good place to start looking for help is your family doctor. Doctors are trained to handle medical problems. Some are especially good at handling persons who are in withdrawal from drugs, including steroids.

Call a doctor at once if you or someone you care about is experiencing any of the following symptoms: nausea or vomiting, spitting up blood, chest pain, blood pressure of 140/90 or over, excessive anger, convulsions, dizziness or fainting, depression, or suicidal thoughts.

Glossary

addict Person who is "hooked" on a drug, or is unable to stop using it.

amphetamines Drugs that excite the mind and body.

anabolic steroids Steroids that build muscle mass.

androgenic steroids Steroids that deepen the voice and cause the growth of facial and body hair and male-pattern baldness.

anhedonia Inability to experience pleasure in normally pleasurable activities.

atrophy To shrink or shrivel up.

black market Illegal trade.

casualty Someone who is injured or killed.

clitoris Small, sensitive tissue at the upper end of the vulva.

corticosteroids Steroids that control inflammation and pain.

diuretic Something that causes the body to rid itself of excess fluid.

doping Drugging athletes or race-horses.

drug abuse Misuse of a drug or use of an illegal drug.

estrogen replacement Use of a synthetic female sex hormone as a replacement for ones that the body has quit producing.

homicidal Tending toward murder.

jaundice Liver disorder.

male-pattern baldness Type of baldness typical in older males.

paranoia Unwarranted suspicion or fear.

prostate gland Gland that surrounds the urethra near its connection to the bladder in the male.

"roid rage" Slang term for the unpredictable, psychotic-like behavior characteristic of some steroid abusers.

testes Male reproductive glands.

testosterone Male sex hormone.

Where to Go For Help

American College of Sports Medicine
P. O. Box 1440
Indianapolis, IN 46206-1440
(317) 637-9200
Web site: http://www.acsm.org/sportsmed

Narcotics Anonymous
19737 Nordhoff Place
Chatsworth, CA 91311
(818) 773-9999
e-mail: wso@aol.com

National Clearinghouse for Alcohol and Drug Information
P. O. Box 2345
Rockville, MD 20847-2345
(301) 468-2600
Web site: http://www.health.org
e-mail: info@prevline.health.org

National Council on Alcoholism and Drug Dependence (NCADD)
12 West 21st Street
New York, NY 10010
(212) 206-6770
(800) 622-2255
Web site: http://www.ncadd.org
e-mail: national@NCADD.org

IN CANADA

Addiction Foundation
(204) 944-6200

Narcotics Anonymous
(416) 691-9519
Web site: http://www.members.better.net/
  toronto_na

Youth Detox Program
Family Services Greater Vancouver
1193 Kingsway, Suite 202
Vancouver, BC V5V 3C9
(604) 872-4349

HOTLINES AND WEB SITES

Al-Anon and Nar-Anon
Hotline: (310) 547-5800

American Self-Help Group Clearing-
  house
Hotline: (973) 625-3037 or (201) 625-9053
Web site: http://www.cmhc.com/selfhelp/

Boys Town National Hotline
Hotline: (800) 448-3000
Web site:http://www.ffbh.boystown.org/
  Hotline/crisis_hotline.htm

60 | **The Center for Substance Abuse Treatment**
Hotline: (800) 662-HELP

Narcotics Anonymous
Hotline: (800) 763-9000
Meeting information: (818) 773-9999
Web site: http://www.wsoinc.com

National Hotline on Alcoholism and Drug Dependence, Inc.
Hotline: (800) NCA-CALL
Web site: http://www.health.org/phone. htm#phone

Substance Abuse Mental Health Services Administration
Drug and Alcohol Treatment Referrals
Hotline: (800) 662-HELP
Web site:
http://www.health.org/phone.htm#phone

For Further Reading

Miklowitz, Gloria D. *Anything to Win.*
   New York: Bantam, Doubleday, Dell,
   1990.
Olinekova, Gayle. *Winning Without
   Steroids.* New Canaan, CT: Keats Pub-
   lishing, 1988.
Peck, Rodney G. *Drugs and Sports.* New
   York: Rosen Publishing Group, 1997.
Rogak, Lisa Angowski. *Steroids: Dangerous
   Game.* Minneapolis, MN: Lerner
   Group, 1992.

Challenging Reading

Taylor, William N. *Anabolic Steroids and
   the Athlete.* Jefferson, NC: McFarland
   & Co., 1982.
——. *Macho Medicine: A History of the*

62 *Anabolic Steroid Epidemic.* Jefferson, NC: McFarland & Co., 1991.

Thomas, J. A. *Drugs, Athletes and Physical Performance.* New York: Plenum, 1988.

Videos
"Anabolic Steroids: The Quest for Superman." Minneapolis: Hourglass Productions, 1990.
"What Price Glory? Myths and Realities of Anabolic Steroids." Edison, NJ: David Thomas Productions, 1989.

Index

About the Author

Lawrence Clayton is an international certified alcohol and drug counselor and president of the Oklahoma Drug and Alcohol Professional Counselor Certification Board. In 1994 he was selected Oklahoma "Counselor of the Year" by the Oklahoma Drug and Alcohol Counselor Association. He lives in Piedmont, Oklahoma, with his wife, Cathy, and their three teenage children.

Photo Credits

p. 15 by Kim Sonsky, pp. 18, 40 © A/P Wide World Photos, p.22 by Guillermina de Ferrari, pp. 51, 54 by Maria Moreno, all other photos and cover by John Novajosky.

CAYUGA COMMUNITY COLLEGE

3 2551 00139321 8

RC
1230   Clayton, L.
.C538
1999   Steroids

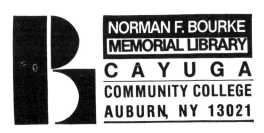
NORMAN F. BOURKE
MEMORIAL LIBRARY
C A Y U G A
COMMUNITY COLLEGE
AUBURN, NY 13021